KETO DESSERTS

COOKBOOK 2019:

THE COMPLETE GUIDE TO A KETOGENIC DESSERT MEAL PLAN, KETO DESSERT COOKBOOK, RECIPES AND GROCERIES FOR SUCCESSFUL WEIGHT LOSS AND OVERAL BODY HEALTH.

BY PHILIP KOCH.

TABLE OF CONTENTS.

WHY YOU SHOULD READ THIS BOOK.................................... 3

INTRODUCTION. 6

Where to find keto desserts. 9

Sugar free sweeteners. 11

TYPES OF KETO DESSERTS FOR YOUR DIET. 14

Homemade keto truffles.. 17

15 BEST KETO DESSERTS OF ALL TIME. 24

WHY YOU SHOULD READ THIS BOOK.

If you are finding a hard time getting the right approach to keto desserts, then it means you are not satisfied with what you have been reading about it.
Desserts are the kind of meals that you can't let go of them easily and this becomes conflicting when getting into keto diet.

Chocolate is the first thing that pops up in your mind whenever you think of a dessert, their mere definition actually involves sweet staff.

In this book, we have compiled all the means of preparing keto desserts which is delicious and it won't make you go crazy about chocolate.

If you are looking for a complete closure about keto dessert and how to prepare some, then you've come to the right place.

If you find this information useful, please leave us a review and we shall be grateful.

INTRODUCTION.

Despite the fact that we are trying to cut down on the carbs, desserts can still fit in even if their mere definition involves sweet staff.

These days its not hard as you think to get yourself a tasty dessert which is 100% keto friendly.

Due to the availability of keto friendly ingredients in the market, you can now make your own desserts and enjoy the ketogenic diet with absolutely no regrets whatsoever.

Finding a ready-made keto friendly dessert on the go isn't an easy task because you cant run into a local grocery store and find an already packaged low carb dessert or snack.

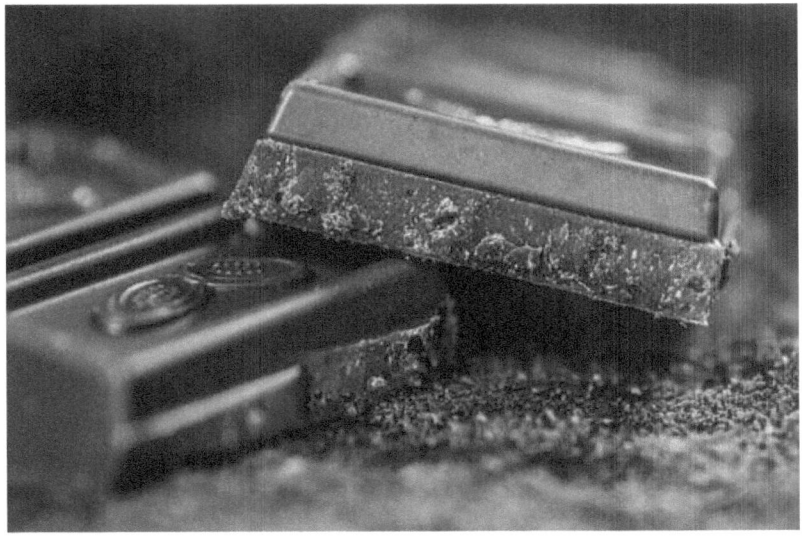

There is always more fun in making your own tasty desserts, something that you are absolutely sure that the ingredients are accurate and not some made up staff on the labels.

Fortunate enough, there is always a way to make keto diet far much less boring.

Just have your alternative sweeteners ready.

Where to find keto desserts.

These days its very much fortunate that the internet makes everything easier.

Whatever you want is just a click away.

Stores dealing with keto foods do the little tasks for you by assembling all the ingredients you want with already calculated macros when we sometimes cant simply make them ourselves.

Some of them are extremely gorgeous, you cant imagine that they are available on the internet pre made.

Better still if you can access a local specialist health grocery store in your area don't hesitate to avail yourself there.

Some of the best ketogenic sweeteners use stevia or erythritol since their impact on glycemic is actually the lowest.

Depending on your specific health needs, you can decide on whether to use any of the above sweeteners or maltitol or xylitol.

These depends on whether you are looking for low carb, sugar free desserts, keto candy or any sweet treats to purchase.

Sugar alcohols are always subtracted from the carb count for keto diet as it has a insignificant impact on blood sugar level.

Always check the nutritional information on the keto desserts bought from the stores but if there isn't some, you can still go read the reviews from other customers and how they feel about the products including the company's Q n A with their customers.

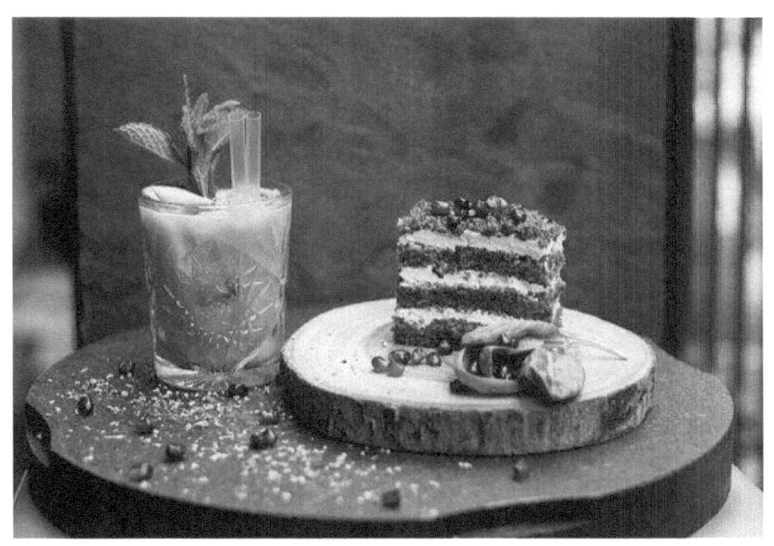

TYPES OF KETO DESSERTS FOR YOUR DIET.

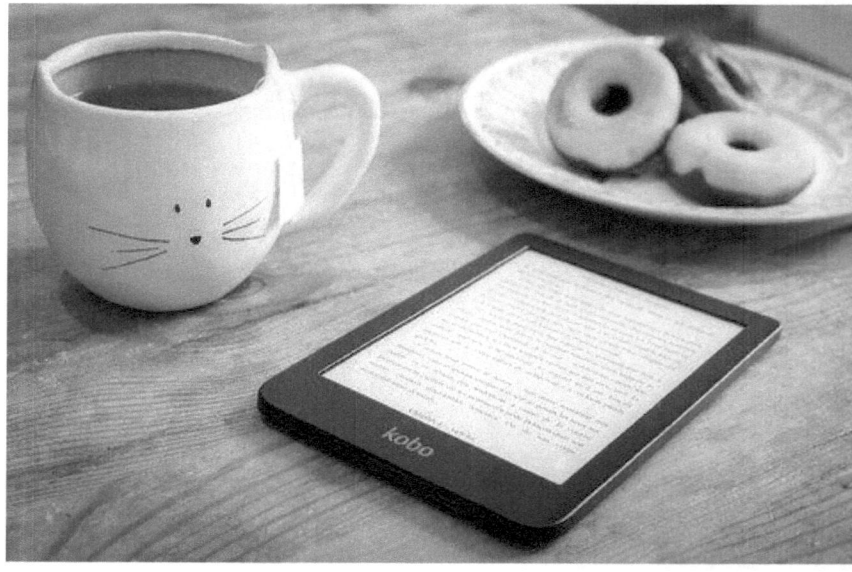

Chocolate dessert always gets bad representation due to its impacts such as causing acne, weight gain and a whole bunch of ailments.

So the big question is if you could possibly have chocolate on keto?

The answer is absolutely yes. It just depends on the macros and the goals you want to achieve.

You can follow the ketogenic lifestyle and enjoy chocolate very well.

The keto chocolate truffles just calls for some ingredients and you can prepare them at the comfort of your home if you can't find them online.

Always use the low carb sweeteners or you can substitute it with erythritol if you cant find powdered monk fruit.

A real chocolate if primarily full of
antioxidants, iron, fiber, fat, magnesium,
manganese and other minerals.

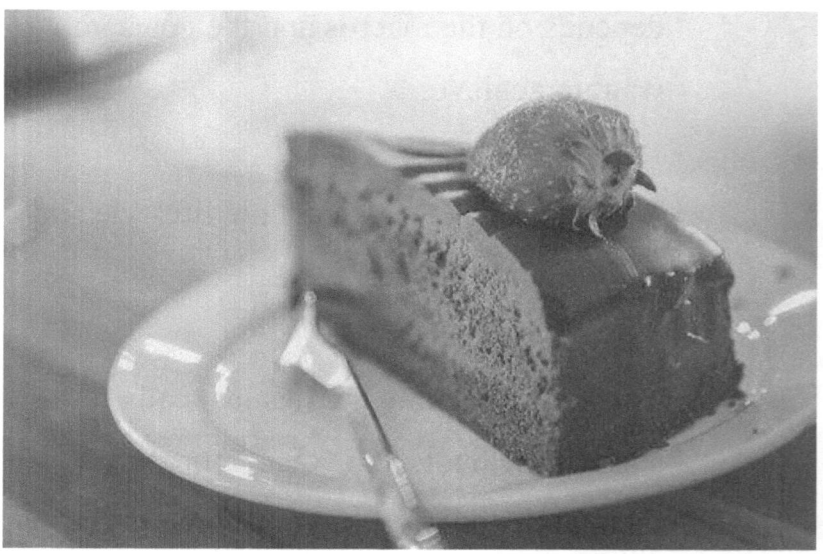

It actually helps improve brain function,
reduce blood pressure among its many
functions.

Homemade keto truffles.

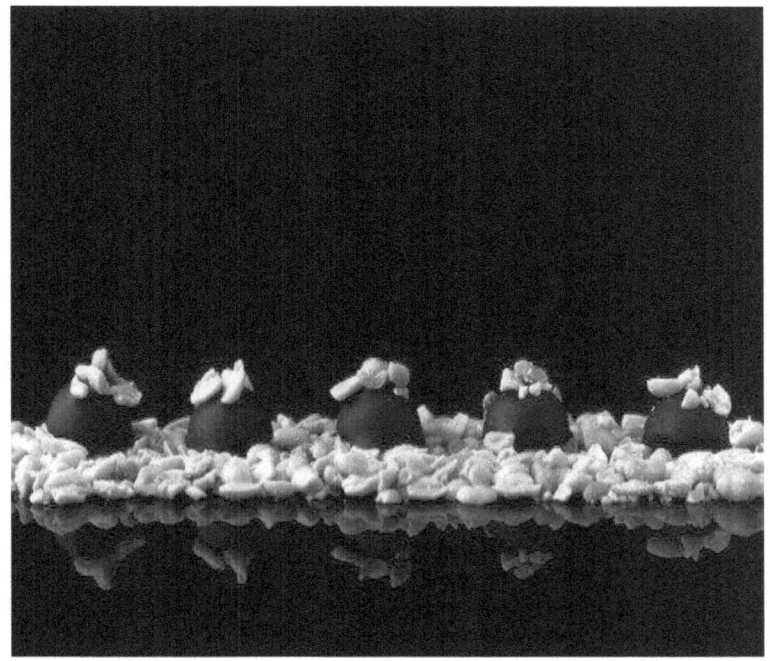

Chocolate.

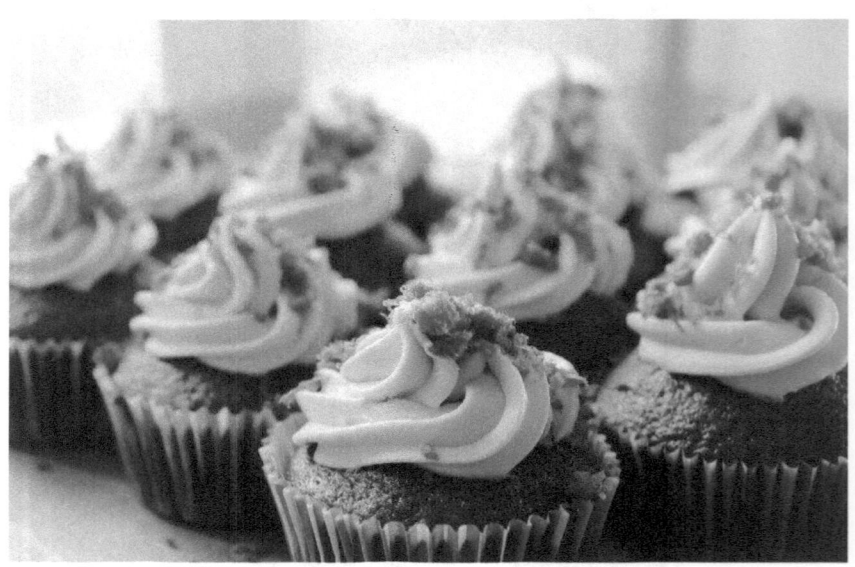

Macros per truffle:

Fat 12g.

Proteins 1.5g.

Carbs 5.5g.

Calories 142g.

The following is a recipe for a dessert serving 12 truffles.

Prep tome is 30 minutes.

Ingredients are as follows.

i. Half cup of heavy cream.
ii. 85% dark chocolate (150g).
iii. 2 tablespoon grass fed butter, 2 tablespoon of honey or any sugar free sweetener.
iv. Half tablespoon of pure vanilla extract.
v. Half tablespoon of cinnamon.

vi.   One pinch of sea salt.

vii.   2 tablespoon of raw cocoa powder.

Procedure.

Heat the cream on a low flame, don't let it boil. Then chop the chocolate bars into small pieces.

As it simmers, add the chopped chocolate to the cream and stir them thoroughly until its combined. While stirring, add the butter until its completely melted.

Stop heating add honey, cinnamon, salt and vanilla, stirr to mix.

Put the mixture in the fridge for an hour.

Remove the mixture from the fridge and scoop some truffle butter and roll them into small balls or to the size you like.

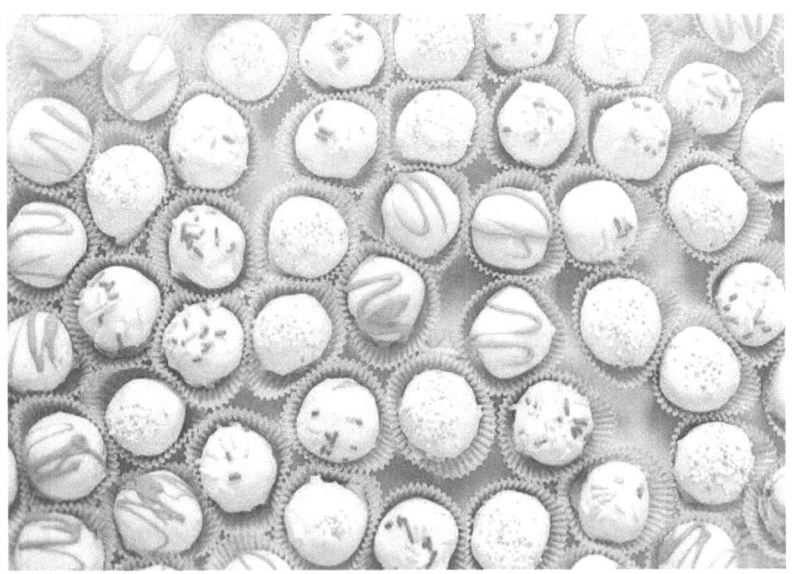

Put the rounded balls on a wax lined plate and refrigerate them for 30 minutes.

Once hardened, add the truffles into a cocoa powder bowl. Shake them gently so that the cocoa powder coat them evenly.

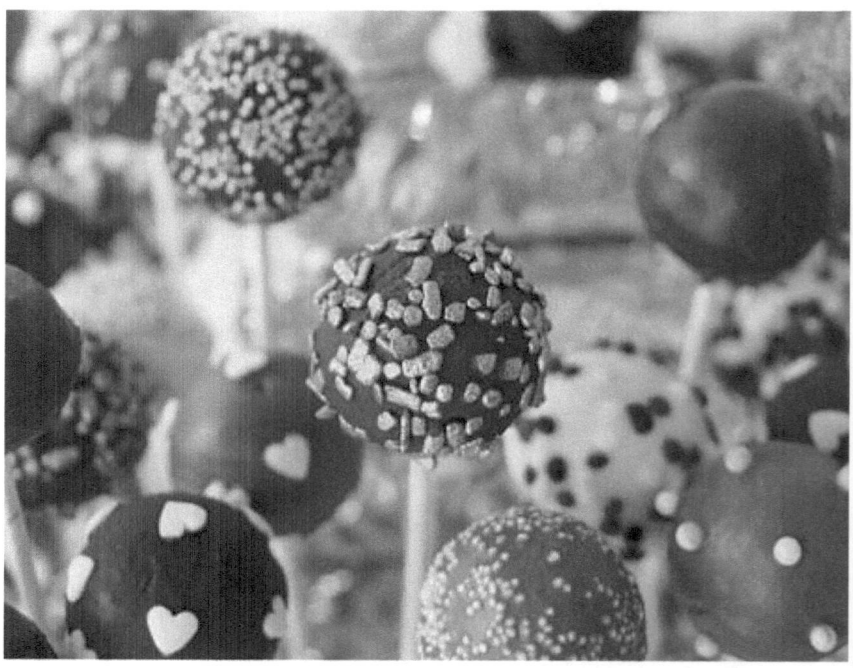

Go ahead and put the truffles in an airtight container until they are ready to serve.

Enjoy them with hot tea.

Whenever you use a sugar free alternative to honey, then be sure to make truffles with even very low carbs.

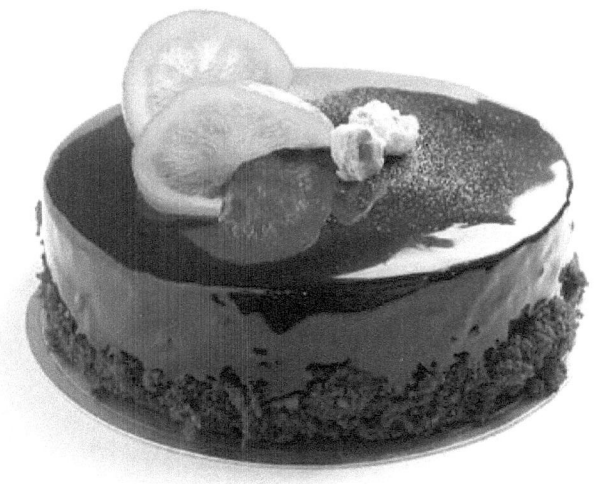

15 BEST KETO DESSERTS OF ALL TIME.

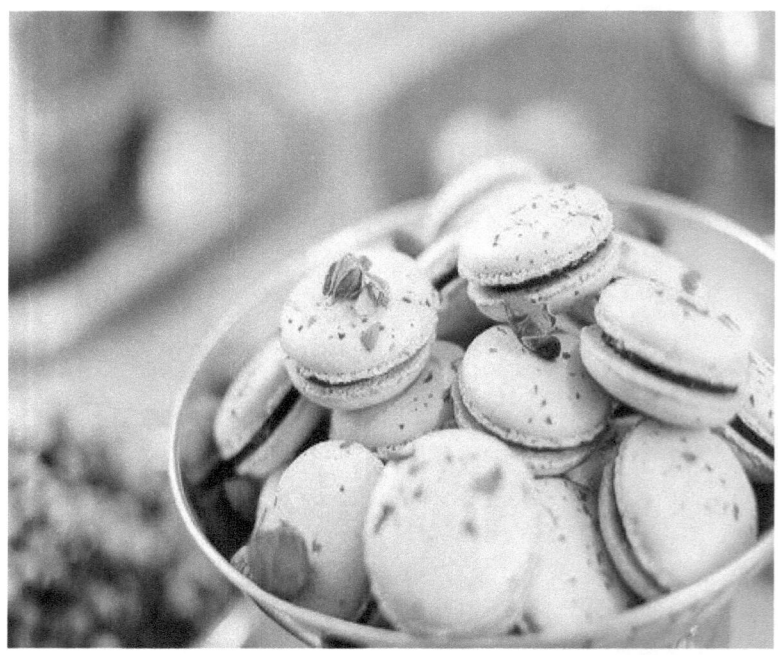

Here are some of the ketogenic desserts that always make the diet better.

So now you are ready to make some dessert by yourself? Okay, grab some keto friendly dark chocolate, alternative sweeteners, nut flours and not forgetting butter.

1) Vanilla pound cake.

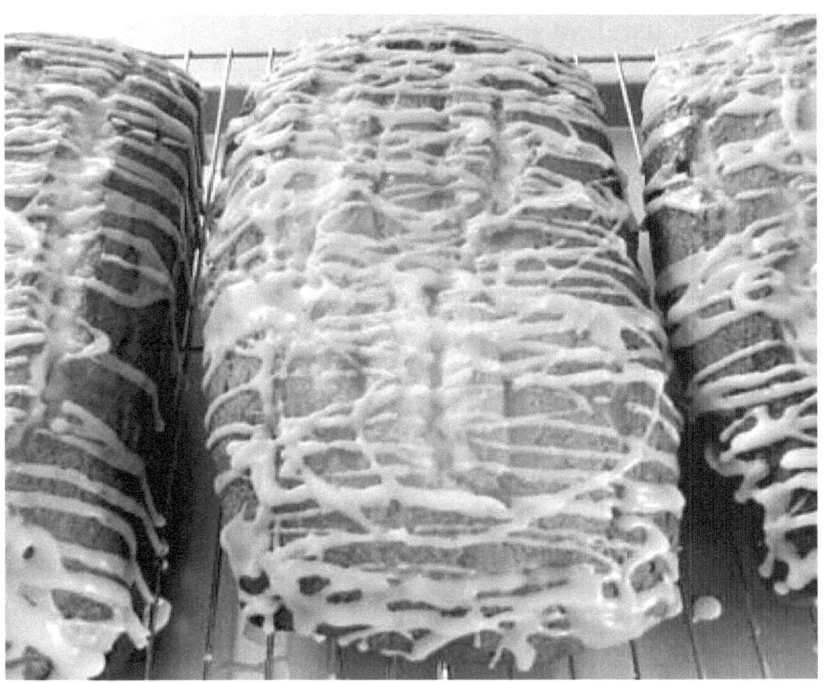

The pound cakes which are usually rich in butter are not likely to be associated with healthy eating.

On the other hand, the eggs and sour cream present in the recipe is comfortably within the ketogenic diet plan.

Crafting the recipe must cut down the carbs by precisely using the almond flour and erythritol which are com-derived and used as sugar alternatives.

2) The vegan coconut macaroons.

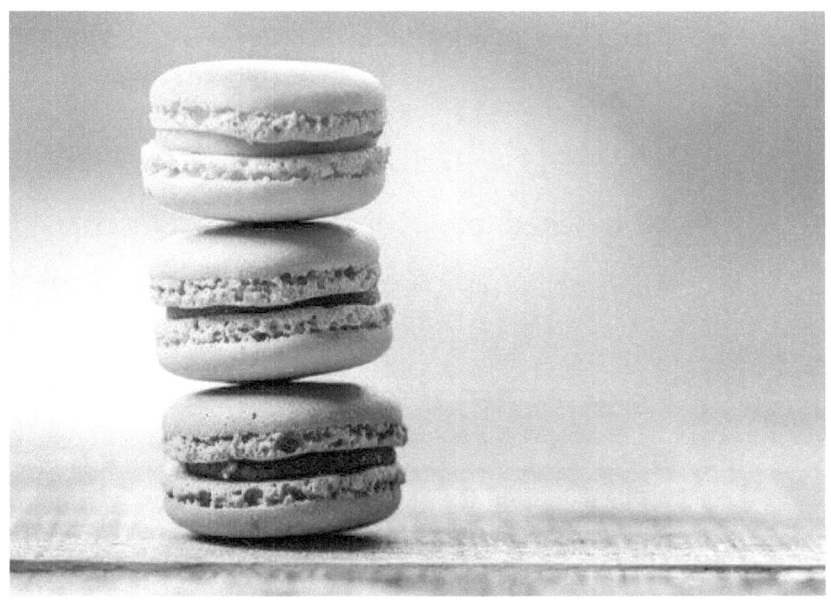

Getting into keto might push you to begin experimenting on the ingredients you never thought of using.

For example the vegan treats are usually held together with a liquid from a can of chickpeas, aquafaba.

But still having the shredded coconut and the smooth chocolate at the bottom can make them have that taste like the usual mouthwatering macaroons you've always loved.

3) Non-baked low carb strawberry lemon cheesecake.

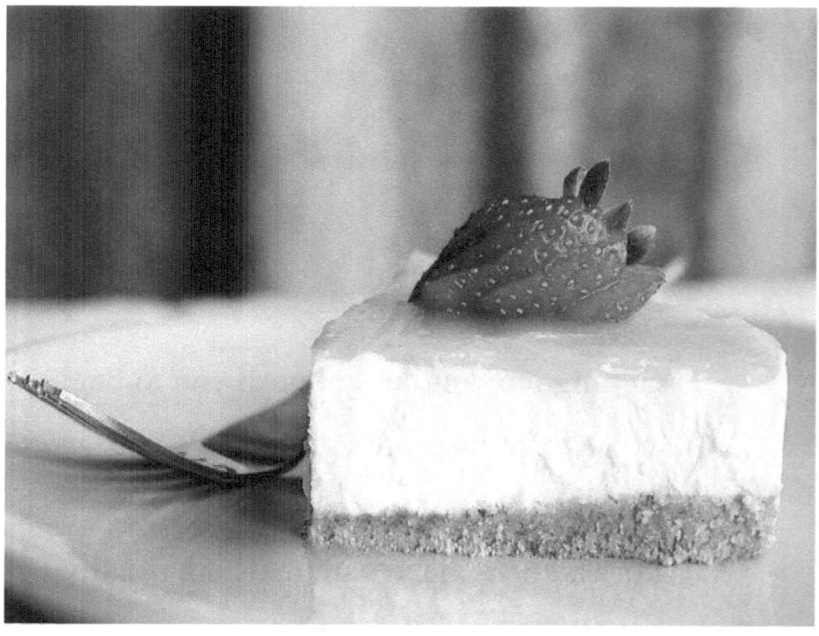

Coming up with this takes the hassle of doing away with the pie crust and this kind of a take on cheesecake goes direct to the point creating layers of sharp strawberries forming a rich cream cheese mixture which is very much refreshing.

4) Orange cake balls.

Use of coconut flour equally replaces the regular ones to keep these cake balls completely ketogenic.
Better still these cakes require no baking at all, it just involves mixing, rolling and enjoy your dish.

5) Maple pecan cheesecake bars.

These have to be grain free.
Sometimes, the plain cheesecake become a bit too bland for you concerning their texture, the recipe for this dessert will help smoothen things up.

Having the powdery almond flour pastry and sprinkling the pecans throughout the filling, can give enough crunch to keep the boredom at a distance.

6) Cocoa butter keto blondies.

With plenty of both regular and the cocoa variety of butter plus eggs and coconut cream, they always turn into a replica of the blondies shape; talk of dense, fudgy and very addictive.
Its not easy to recognize the difference even if you give to a non keto people, they won't notice.

7) Butter pecan ice cream.

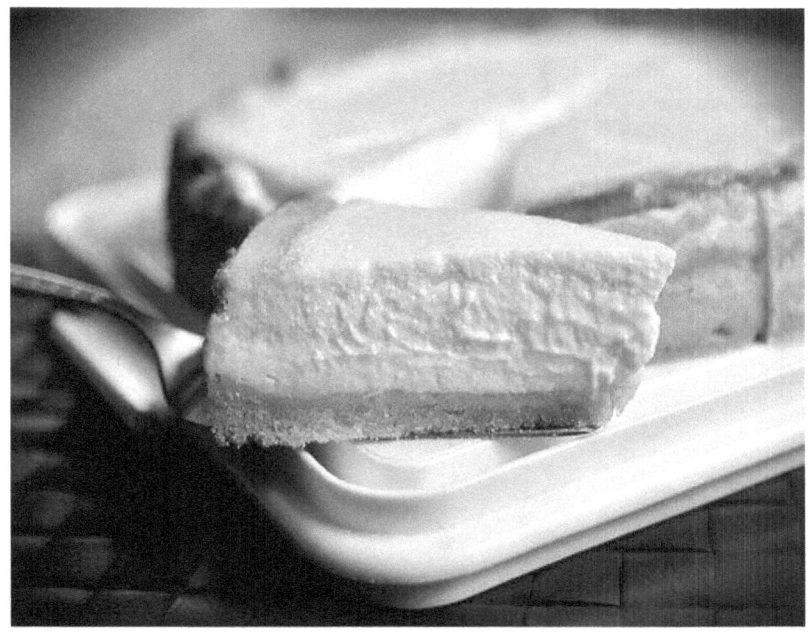

This totally doesn't require an ice cream machine as it can be made in a food processor and just freezing in a loaf pan. This keto ice cream tastes very close to the standard butter pecan scoops you can get.

8) Keto carrot cake.

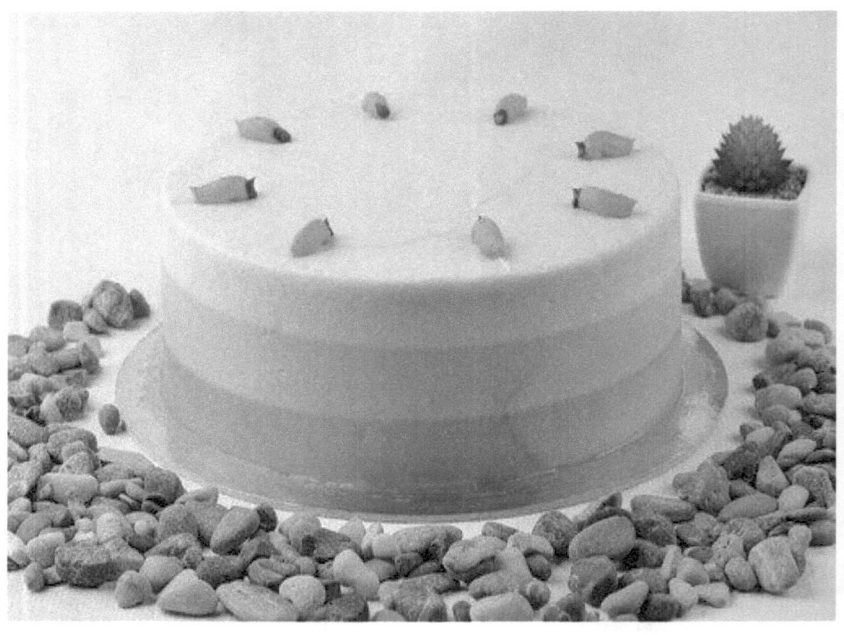

The recipe for this one is actually not so different from that of the regular carrot cake only that you have to add the cream cheese frosting to your ingredients.

9) Pumpkin cheesecake mouse.

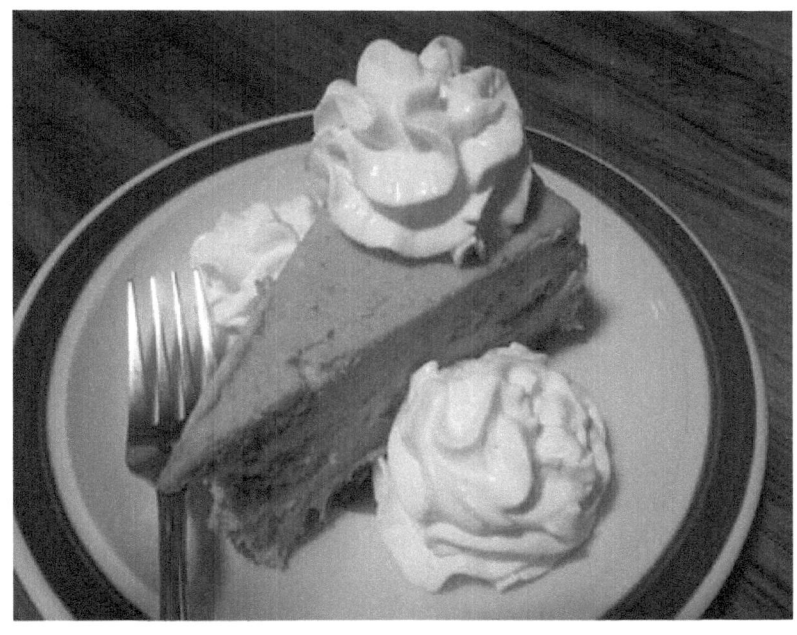

Get yourself some real pumpkin, cook them very well then add some water and stir it into some whipped cheesecake. This will give it some depth and flavor. This mixture is definitely the tastiest source of fiber.

10)   Lemon bars.

If you are in for great fruitiness with absolutely no carbs, then depending on your choice of either battery, zesty or dense, keto lemon bars are your choice.

11)   Avocado brownies.

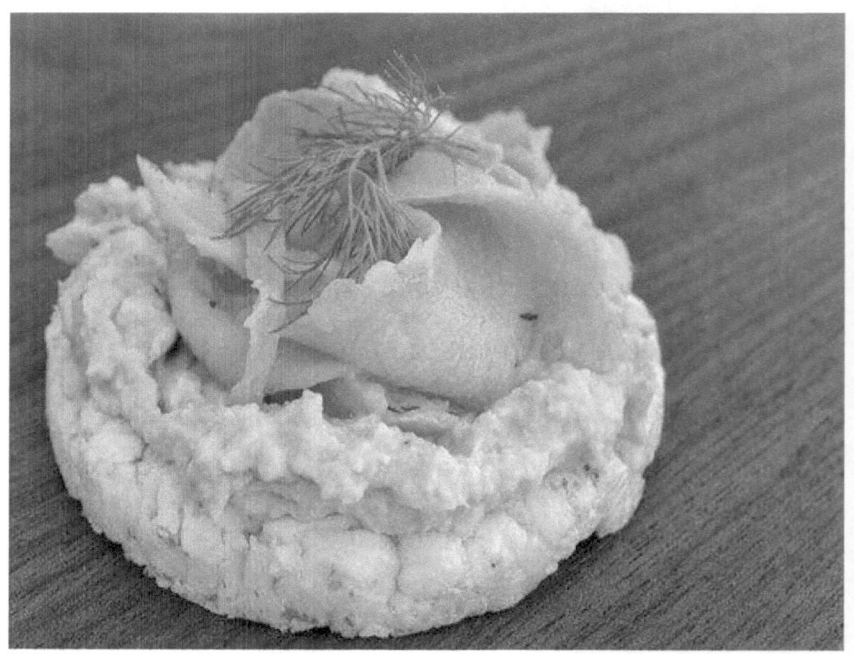

Butter free is the main concern about keto.

Trading off with avocado makes them very much suitable for anybody who likes dairy free dessert

12)   Coconut mocha donuts.

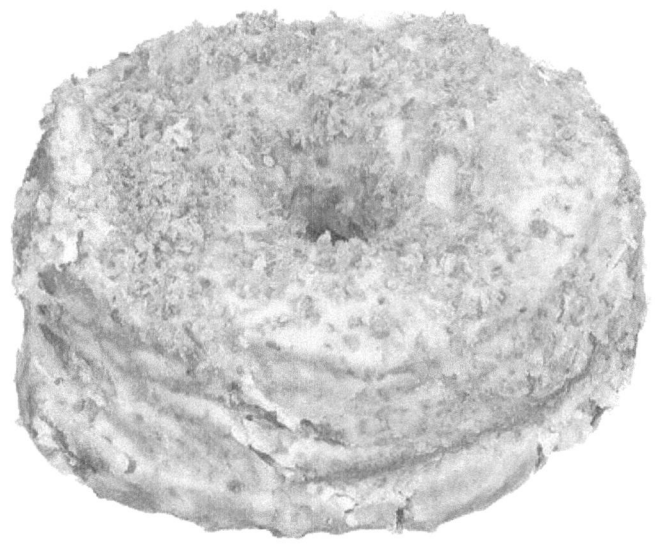

This is the part of the dessert round up with coffee in them.
They are usually packaged with the most satisfying ingredients like eggs, coconut

oil and fiber rich coconut oil. You can therefore enjoy them in the morning too.

13)   Almond joy chia seed pudding.

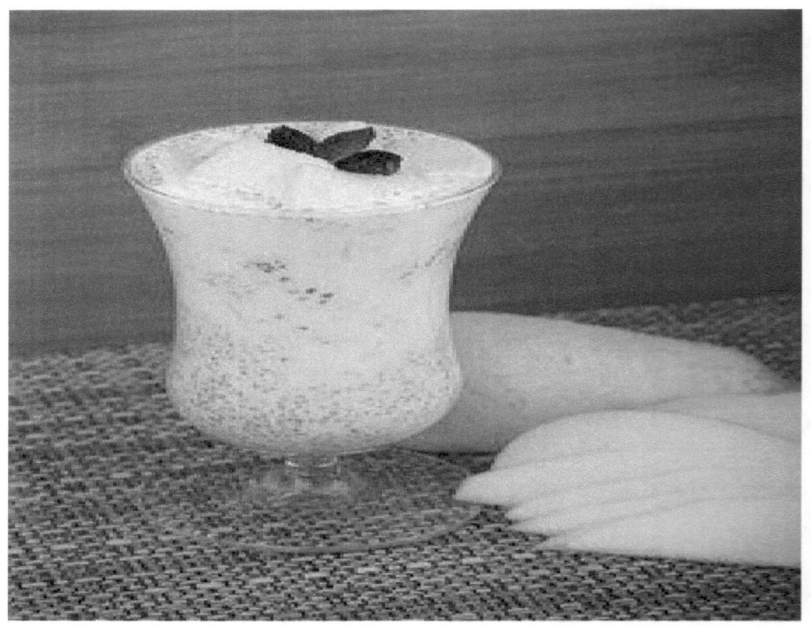

Chia pudding is actually a popular breakfast meal, but on addition of dark chocolate and cocoa powder it automatically qualifies it or a dessert.

14)   Low carb rum balls.

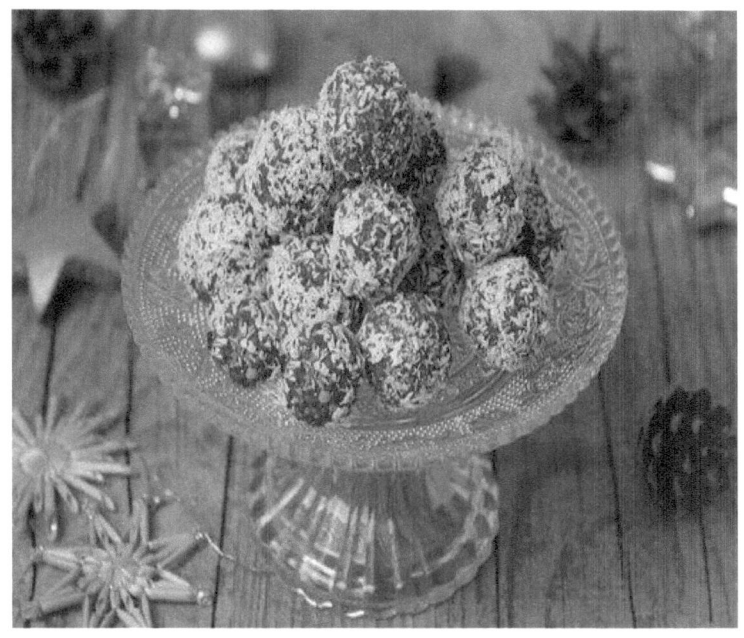

The definitely make you worry less about the sugary treats anytime during the holiday.

15) Sugar free chocolate.

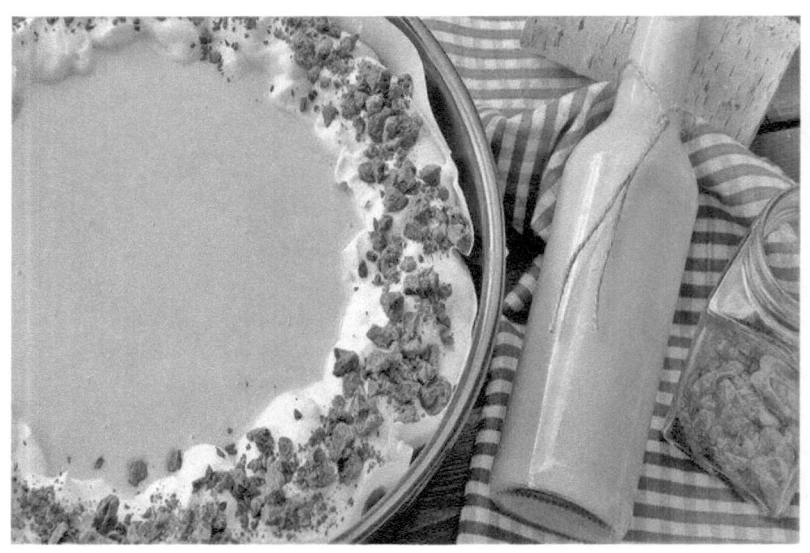

They contain the bacon and almonds.
You will probably love this one since it
requires only 3 ingredients and no ovens
as its easy to prepare.

www.ingramcontent.com/pod-product-compliance
Lightning Source LLC
Chambersburg PA
CBHW061232280526
45784CB00006B/2731